Unlocking the Power of Protein: How the Right Proteins Can Transform Your Health

TABLE OF CONTENT

INTRODUCTION   6

CHAPTER 1: PROTEIN BASICS: UNDERSTANDING THE ROLES OF PROTEIN IN THE BODY   8

What Are Proteins and What Are They Made Of?   8

The Many Roles of Proteins   9

Essential vs Non-essential Amino Acids   10

Protein Digestion and Absorption   10

CHAPTER 2: SIGNS AND CONSEQUENCES OF PROTEIN DEFICIENCY   12

What Causes Protein Deficiency?   12

Symptoms and Health Risks   13

Hidden Signs of Deficiency   14

CHAPTER 3: PROTEIN QUALITY MATTERS   16

What Makes a Protein Source "High Quality"?   16

Complete vs Incomplete Proteins   17

Evaluating Protein Quality by PDCAAS   18

Comparing Whey, Casein, Soy, Pea and Other Proteins   19

How Preparation and Processing Affects Quality   20

CHAPTER 4: HARNESSING THE POWER OF PROTEIN FOR WEIGHT LOSS   21

The Exceptional Satiating Power of Protein   21

Preserving or Building Lean Muscle Mass 22

Protein's Metabolic Advantage and Thermogenic Effect 23

Sample High Protein Meal Plans 23

Tracking and Adjusting Protein Intake 24

CHAPTER 5: PROTEIN FOR ENERGY, PERFORMANCE AND RECOVERY 26

Protein Provides Sustained Energy 26

Pre- and Post-Workout Protein Recommendations 27

Maximizing Amino Acid Availability and Uptake 28

Protein Timing for Strength vs Endurance Athletes 29

Protein for Faster Recovery 29

CHAPTER 6: PROTEIN FOR IMMUNITY, BONE HEALTH, AND DISEASE PREVENTION 31

Protein Supports Immune Function 31

Protein for Bone Health 32

Protein and Longevity 32

Protein Defends Against Metabolic Disease 33

Protein's Antioxidant and Anti-Inflammatory Effects 34

CHAPTER 7: FINDING YOUR PROTEIN SWEET SPOT 36

How Much Protein Do You Need? 36

Signs You May Need More Protein 37

Signs You Need Less Protein 38

Fine Tuning Your Intake   38

Incorporating Quality Protein Sources   39

CONCLUSION   40

Start Unlocking Protein's Potential   41

Parting Words   42

ABOUT THE AUTHOR   43

Introduction

Proteins are essential compounds that play a critical role in nearly all biological processes in the human body. From enzymes that catalyze chemical reactions, to antibodies that recognize and fight pathogens, to structural components like collagen and keratin, proteins perform a staggeringly diverse array of functions that are absolutely vital for life.

Despite their importance, many people do not give much thought to their daily protein intake. The Recommended Dietary Allowance (RDA) for protein is a modest 0.8 grams per kilogram of body weight per day. However, evidence suggests that the RDA may not be adequate for optimal health and disease prevention, especially as we age. Studies show that inadequate protein intake can negatively impact muscle mass, bone density, satiety and weight management, athletic performance, immune function, and recovery from illness or injury.

Emerging research indicates that making smart protein choices may provide profound benefits extending well beyond the commonly recognized sports and fitness goals. Higher protein diets have been associated with increased lifespan, reduced cardiovascular risk factors, improved body composition, healthier aging and reduced risk of age-related muscle loss. Not all proteins are created equal however, and protein quality as determined by digestibility and amino acid content can make a big difference.

This book will take you through everything you need to know about proteins - from how they work in the body, to what constitutes a high-quality protein source, to practical strategies for optimizing your individual protein intake for maximum health and longevity. Backed by the latest scientific evidence, it will address common myths and misconceptions about proteins while uncovering how strategic protein intake can help unlock your full physical and mental potential.

Whether your goals are muscular strength, fat loss, injury recovery, improved immunity or simply healthy aging, the right proteins can transform your health. This book will be your guide to understanding protein needs for different goals, identifying high-quality protein sources that work for your lifestyle and budget, timing protein intake, designing balanced high protein meals, and tracking and adjusting your protein consumption. You will learn actionable best practices for harnessing the proven benefits of protein.

Armed with evidence-based protein wisdom, you will have the knowledge needed to tailor your diet and transform your health for the better. Let's get started unlocking the incredible power of protein!

Chapter 1: Protein Basics: Understanding the Roles of Protein in the Body

Proteins are one of the fundamental macronutrients that make life possible. The human body contains over 10,000 different proteins, each with a specific structure and function. In this chapter, we will cover:

- What proteins are and their chemical structure

- The diverse roles proteins play in the body

- Essential and non-essential amino acids

- How proteins are digested and absorbed

Understanding these protein basics will provide context on why sufficient protein intake is crucial for optimal health at every stage of life.

What Are Proteins and What Are They Made Of?

Proteins are large, complex molecules made up of smaller subunits called amino acids. Amino acids are organic compounds that contain amine and carboxyl functional groups. There are 20 different amino acids that combine in varying sequences to form the diverse array of proteins needed for human life.

The sequence and number of amino acids ultimately determine the shape and function of each protein. Short chains of amino acids are called peptides, while longer chains are proteins. The specific three-dimensional structure of a protein is key to enabling it to perform its biological role.

Amino acids link together via peptide bonds to form polypeptide chains. These chains then fold into complex three-dimensional protein structures. The sequence of amino acids dictates the folding patterns and final shape of each protein.

The Many Roles of Proteins

The thousands of different proteins in the body have a staggering diversity of critical roles. Here are just some of the vital functions proteins perform:

- **Enzymes** - Catalyze and accelerate chemical reactions in the body

- **Messenger proteins** - Transmit signals between cells and tissues

- **Transport proteins** - Carry molecules like oxygen through the bloodstream

- **Structural proteins** - Provide structure and support e.g. collagen, keratin

- **Storage proteins** - Store and supply amino acids when needed

- **Hormones** - Coordinate growth, metabolism and other systems

- **Antibodies** - Identify and neutralize pathogens like bacteria and viruses

- **Motor proteins** - Enable muscle contraction

- **Clotting factors** - Assist in blood clotting

In essence, proteins participate in every physiological process needed to sustain life. Sufficient intake of the right proteins is crucial for maintaining health. Shortfalls can negatively impact countless aspects of health and function.

Essential vs Non-essential Amino Acids

Of the 20 amino acids needed to build proteins, 9 are considered essential amino acids. They are labeled essential because the body cannot produce them endogenously - we can only obtain them through diet. The 9 essential amino acids are:

- Histidine

- Isoleucine

- Leucine

- Lysine

- Methionine

- Phenylalanine

- Threonine

- Tryptophan

- Valine

The remaining 11 amino acids are non-essential, meaning they can be synthesized by the body as needed. However, just because the body can make non-essential amino acids doesn't mean consuming dietary sources is unimportant. Getting adequate amounts from both essential and non-essential amino acids is vital for good health.

Each of the 20 amino acids has distinct properties and influences specific metabolic functions. Amino acid balance and variety is just as important as overall protein quantity. High quality protein sources provide essential and non-essential amino acids in optimal ratios.

Protein Digestion and Absorption

In order for the body to utilize dietary protein, it must first be broken down through digestion into individual amino acids or di- and tri-peptides that can be absorbed.

Digestion begins in the stomach where protein is denatured by stomach acid, uncoiling its complex structure. The protein molecules are then further broken down into smaller polypeptides by pepsin and hydrochloric acid.

As food moves into the small intestine, the pancreas releases proteolytic enzymes like trypsin and chymotrypsin to further cleave polypeptides into individual amino acids. The amino acids and small peptides can then be transported across the intestinal wall into circulation.

The rate of protein digestion and amino acid absorption is influenced by factors like protein source, cooking method, and other foods eaten at the same time. Once amino acids enter the bloodstream, the body utilizes them as needed to build and repair tissue or synthesizes new glucose or fat for energy production.

Now that you understand what proteins are made of, the many roles they serve, and how they are digested - let's move on to the health consequences that can occur if we don't get adequate amounts of the right proteins.

Chapter 2: Signs and Consequences of Protein Deficiency

Not consuming enough high-quality protein can negatively impact nearly every aspect of health and function. However, the signs of protein deficiency can sometimes be subtle or non-specific, making it hard to recognize. In this chapter we will cover:

- What causes protein deficiency

- The symptoms and health risks linked to low protein intake

- Hidden signs you may not be getting enough protein

Understanding the many consequences of protein deficiency, even mild cases, highlights why sufficient daily protein is so important. Catching warnings signs early on allows you to adjust intake before health impacts snowball.

What Causes Protein Deficiency?

Protein deficiency can stem from a variety of factors:

- **Inadequate total calories** - Consuming too few calories to support protein needs

- **Low protein diets** - Follow diets very low in protein sources

- **Malabsorption issues** - Conditions like IBD or celiac impede protein absorption

- **Medications** - Certain drugs increase protein requirement

- **Increased needs** - Growing children, pregnancy, athletes need more

- **Age-related anorexia** - Appetite and intake often decline with age

Vegans and vegetarians can also be at risk if not carefully meeting protein needs from plant sources. Even omnivores who eat a standard Western diet can have low grade protein deficiency due to excessive processing and calorie intake skewed toward carbs and fats rather than protein.

Symptoms and Health Risks

The most overt symptom of severe protein deficiency is muscle wasting and loss of lean mass as the body breaks down tissue to salvage amino acids. However, long before this stage, moderate protein deficiency can have many consequences:

- **Impaired immune function** - Lack of amino acids to build antibodies

- **Delayed growth and developmental milestones in children**

- **Loss of muscle mass and decreased strength**

- **Fat gain and distorted body composition** - Body cannibalizes muscle for energy

- **Hormone imbalance** - Amino acids needed to synthesize key hormones

- **Low energy and endurance** - Inability to produce glucose between meals

- **Mood issues and trouble concentrating** - Lack of amino acid precursors for neurotransmitters

- **Poor wound healing and long recovery from illness/injury**

- **Higher risk of bone fractures** - Inadequate protein undermines bone matrix

- **Greater risk of metabolic syndrome and type 2 diabetes**

As you can see, even marginal protein deficiency takes a toll on health in myriad ways. Let's now look at hidden signs of low protein intake.

Hidden Signs of Deficiency

Overt protein deficiency with pronounced muscle wasting is rare in developed nations. However, chronic low grade deficiency can still exist and negatively impact health in subtle ways. Here are some hidden signs of inadequate protein intake:

- **Constant hunger and cravings** - Body seeks amino acids needed for tissue repair

- **High BMI but low muscle mass** - Lean mass is cannibalized despite excess fat

- **Frequent injuries and slow healing** - Lack of amino acids to rebuild tissue

- **Thinning hair or brittle nails** - Lack of amino acids for keratin

- **Foggy thinking and trouble concentrating** - Need protein to produce alertness chemicals

- **Unrestful sleep** - Amino acid imbalance disrupts sleep hormones

- **Low libido and sexual dysfunction** - Protein important for sex hormone balance

- **Susceptibility to frequent colds/infections** - Protein vital for immune function

- **Slow recovery from exercise** - Protein needed for muscle repair and rebuilding

Paying attention to these potential signals of inadequate protein allows you to address deficits through diet before health impacts grow more severe.

Now that you understand the diverse roles protein plays in the body, recognize warning signs of deficiency, and appreciate why sufficient daily protein matters - let's move on to discussing optimal protein quality and sources.

Chapter 3: Protein Quality Matters

When it comes to protein foods, quality matters just as much, if not more than quantity. Some proteins are more efficiently digested, absorbed and utilized than others. Understanding what makes a protein "high quality" allows you to make optimal choices. We will cover:

- Defining high quality protein

- Complete vs incomplete proteins

- Evaluating protein quality by PDCAAS score

- Comparing common proteins like whey, soy, casein, pea etc.

- How preparation and processing affects protein quality

Appreciating key differences in protein quality empowers you to maximize the nutritional value you derive from your protein choices.

What Makes a Protein Source "High Quality"?

The quality of a protein source refers to its ability to provide adequate amounts of the essential amino acids in ratios that can be efficiently used by the body.

Several factors determine protein quality:

- **Digestibility** - How easily the protein can be broken down into amino acids during digestion. Proteins that are easily digested and absorbed are higher quality.

- **Essential amino acid content** - A complete protein contains all 9 essential amino acids in sufficient quantities. Incomplete

proteins are low in or missing one or more essential amino
acids.

- **Amino acid profile** - The ratios of essential amino acids and
  non-essential amino acids should match the body's needs.

- **PDCAAS score** - Protein Digestibility Corrected Amino
  Acid Score rates quality from 0-1 based on human
  requirements. Higher is better.

When it comes to protein foods:

- **Animal sources** like eggs, dairy and meat are complete high
  quality proteins.

- **Plant sources** like beans, grains and nuts are often
  incomplete proteins. Combining complementary plant
  proteins can form a complete protein profile.

- **Supplemental proteins** like whey and casein are highly
  digestible with excellent PDCAAS scores near 1.0.

Complete vs Incomplete Proteins

Complete proteins contain all 9 essential amino acids. Most animal
foods like meat, fish, poultry, eggs and dairy are complete proteins.

Plant foods are often incomplete - low or missing one or more
essential amino acids. For example:

- Beans are low in methionine and cysteine

- Grains are low in lysine

- Nuts and seeds lack lysine and threonine

By combining complementary plant proteins like beans and rice, you
can fill in the gaps to form a complete protein. This is the premise
behind dishes like dal and rice or peanut butter sandwiches.

Animal proteins provide the full array of essential amino acids
without the need to complement. For vegans/vegetarians focused

plant-based diets, being mindful of protein combining is important to avoid deficiency.

Now let's look at how the PDCAAS system evaluates protein quality:

Evaluating Protein Quality by PDCAAS

The Protein Digestibility Corrected Amino Acid Score (PDCAAS) is the preferred method for assessing protein quality based on human requirements.

The PDCAAS rates proteins on a 0-1 scale using two key criteria:

1. Digestibility - How readily the protein can be digested and absorbed

2. Essential amino acid content - How closely the protein matches the essential amino acid profile required by humans

For example:

- Egg white protein has a PDCAAS of 1.0 - the highest score. It is highly digestible and provides an optimal amino acid ratio.

- Soy protein has a score of around 0.9. It has good digestibility and amino acid profile but is somewhat deficient in methionine.

- Wheat protein comes in at 0.25-0.5 since it has poor digestibility and lacks some essential amino acids like lysine.

As a general guide:

- 0.9-1.0 = Excellent quality

- 0.7-0.9 = Good quality

- Below 0.7 = Low quality

The PDCAAS scale allows objective comparisons between protein sources to inform choices. Next let's see how it applies to evaluating specific proteins.

Comparing Whey, Casein, Soy, Pea and Other Proteins

Thanks to the PDCAAS system, we can objectively rate the quality of common dietary proteins:

Whey protein - PDCAAS 0.9-1.0

Derived from milk, whey is very high in branched chain amino acids like leucine. It has excellent digestibility and amino acid balance.

Casein protein - PDCAAS 1.0

The other milk protein, casein is high in glutamine and casomorphins that aid digestion. Also highly bioavailable.

Soy protein - PDCAAS 0.9-1.0

Soy is a complete plant protein but lower in methionine. Processed soy has higher PDCAAS than unfermented soybeans.

Pea protein - PDCAAS 0.7-0.8

Pea is deficient in cysteine and methionine but high in lysine. Works well blended with rice protein.

Hemp protein - PDCAAS 0.7-0.8

Hemp is complete but has lower digestibility. High in fiber and omega-3s.

Rice protein - PDCAAS 0.2-0.8

Rice is very low in lysine but high in cysteine and methionine. Can complement legume proteins.

Beef protein - PDCAAS 0.92

Beef is high quality complete protein. Less digestible than whey or egg protein.

This comparison shows how proteins from both plant and animal sources can vary in quality, so being choosy really pays off.

How Preparation and Processing Affects Quality

Preparation methods can alter protein quality. Raw egg whites contain avidin which binds biotin and reduces absorption. Cooking denatures avidin.

Processing can damage protein structure through heating and oxidation, reducing digestibility. Excessive heat treatment of milk protein can decrease its quality.

Sprouting, fermenting and partially pre-digesting plant proteins using enzymes or bacteria can break down antinutrients and make amino acids more bioavailable.

Overall, opting for minimally processed proteins helps preserve quality. With a grasp on what makes a protein "high quality", let's now explore how to strategically leverage protein's power for fat loss...

Chapter 4: Harnessing the Power of Protein for Weight Loss

Obesity has reached epidemic proportions worldwide. Losing excess body fat improves not just appearance but also metabolic health and disease risk. Unfortunately, the vast majority of diets fail in the long run. Strategically harnessing the power of protein may be the key to sustainable weight loss. This chapter will cover:

- Protein's exceptional satiating power

- How protein preserves or builds calorie-burning lean muscle

- The thermogenic effect - protein's metabolic advantage

- Sample high protein meal plans for weight management

- Tracking protein intake for fat loss goals

Understanding protein's unique properties provides a blueprint for utilizing it intelligently to drop fat without sacrificing nutrition or muscle mass.

The Exceptional Satiating Power of Protein

A food's satiating power refers to how satisfying it is - how well it wards off hunger and curbs cravings. Protein is the most satiating macronutrient. Research shows high protein foods lead to:

- **Earlier meal termination** - You automatically eat less calories

- **Delayed subsequent eating** - Increased time till next meal

- **Reduced late night snacking** - Better appetite control

Reasons protein provides exceptional satiety include:

- Requires extensive digestion - Leads to prolonged release of gut satiety hormones

- Elicits a strong insulin response which controls blood sugar and hunger

- Metabolized slower than carbs, providing steady energy and stable blood sugar

- Dense in nutrients like iron needed for optimal appetite regulation

High protein diets enhance satiety and compliance compared to standard low protein weight loss diets. Let's examine specific ways protein aids fat loss.

Preserving or Building Lean Muscle Mass

Diets low in protein cause muscle loss rather than just fat reduction. Muscle is metabolically active and burns more calories than fat - it's crucial for maintaining a robust metabolism.

Adequate protein intake preserves lean muscle mass as you drop fat by:

- Providing amino acid building blocks to maintain muscle tissue

- Supporting muscle protein synthesis to build and strengthen muscle

- Slowing muscle protein breakdown during weight loss

Higher protein also helps build more lean muscle. Resistance exercise coupled with sufficient protein stimulates muscle protein synthesis. The amino acid leucine is especially important, spiking muscle growth via mTOR activation.

A University of Illinois study evaluating obese dieters found that those consuming 1.2 g of protein per kg of body weight preserved more lean muscle and lost more fat than those eating only 0.8 g/kg. Protein quantity really matters when cutting calories for fat loss.

Protein's Metabolic Advantage and Thermogenic Effect

Protein provides a metabolic advantage driving fat burning. The thermic effect of food refers to the energy expended digesting and metabolizing nutrients. Of all the macronutrients, protein has by far the highest thermic effect - 20-35% of protein's calories are burned during digestion and use.

Reasons protein has a sky-high thermic effect include:

- Extensive breakdown into amino acids

- Activation of urea cycle to dispose of nitrogen byproduct

- High ATP cost of peptide bond synthesis

- Synthesis of protein-related molecules like glutathione

    Clinical studies find substituting protein for fat and carbs significantly increases total energy expenditure. Boosting protein to 30% of calories can upregulate body fat oxidation by 80%. Thermogenesis makes higher protein intake ideal for weight loss.

Sample High Protein Meal Plans

To leverage protein's exceptional satiety and fat burning properties, meals plans for weight loss should provide:

- **0.6-1 g protein per lb ideal body weight** This preserves lean mass while cutting fat. For a 150 lb goal weight, target 90-150 g protein daily.

- **Protein evenly distributed at meals and snacks** Spreading out protein stabilizes blood sugar and mTOR activation for consistent satiety and muscle building.

- **30% of calories from protein** Increased protein with modest fat (30%) and lower refined carbs optimizes thermogenesis.

Here's a sample high protein day with 30% calories from protein:

Breakfast - Scrambled eggs (18 g protein) with veggies

Snack - Nonfat Greek yogurt (15 g) with berries

Lunch - Grilled chicken (30 g) salad with chickpeas (7 g)

Snack - Lowfat cottage cheese (15 g) and raw almonds (8 g)

Dinner - Salmon (25 g), quinoa (4 g) and asparagus

Evening Snack - Whey protein shake (25 g)

This provides 150 g of protein split evenly into 30+ gram doses spaced throughout the day along with ample fiber and nutrients.

Let's look at tracking protein intake for fat loss goals...

Tracking and Adjusting Protein Intake

To dial in adequate protein intake for weight management, tracking intake using a food journal, app or macros tracker is recommended. Here are key steps:

1. **Determine ideal body weight protein target** 0.6 - 1 g per lb ideal weight. Err on the higher side if very active.

2. **Track protein grams consumed for 3-5 days** Include all food, beverages and supplements.

3. **Compare average intake to target protein amount** Is current protein below, at, or above the goal range?

4. **Adjust daily protein intake gradually** If below target, add 10-20 g by incorporating more lean proteins, protein supplements, or high protein versions of foods you eat regularly. Reassess weekly.

5. **Time protein distribution** Aim for minimum 25-30 g protein at each meal, 15-20 g per snack.

Fine tuning protein consumption while tracking macros and body weight empowers you to achieve fat loss goals and retain lean muscle in a sustainable way.

Chapter 5: Protein for Energy, Performance and Recovery

Protein plays key roles in physical performance and recovery. Well-trained athletes have higher protein needs to support their activity levels and strength building goals. Strategically timing quality proteins around workouts also optimizes gains. This chapter will cover:

- Protein and sustained energy production

- Pre- and post-workout protein recommendations

- Maximizing amino acid availability and uptake

- Protein timing for strength athletes vs endurance athletes

- Optimizing protein intake for faster recovery

Harnessing protein's performance-enhancing and recuperative powers allows you to reach new levels of athletic achievement.

Protein Provides Sustained Energy

Carbohydrates serve as the primary fuel powering high intensity exercise. However, carbs only maintain blood glucose and energy for about 2 hours - then glycogen stores deplete triggering fatigue. This is where protein steps in to take over...

Dietary protein is broken down into amino acids that can in turn be converted into glucose via gluconeogenesis. This provides a steady supply of glucose into the bloodstream to power muscles.

With adequate protein intake, gluconeogenesis can contribute up to 10% of the total energy utilized during prolonged endurance exercise. This helps counteract glycogen depletion and delays fatigue.

During strength training, protein-derived glucose aids performance by:

- Sparing muscle glycogen

- Supporting muscle contraction

- Enhancing resistance to fatigue

Clearly protein provides unique energetic advantages. Optimizing intake around exercise is important.

Pre- and Post-Workout Protein Recommendations

Bookending workouts with protein helps amplify gains. The main goals are to:

- Provide amino acids to minimize muscle damage and accelerate repair

- Spike protein synthesis for muscle growth

- Restore depleted glycogen stores

Pre-workout protein is beneficial to:

- Supply amino acids to muscles before exertion

- Increase blood flow and nutrient delivery to muscles

- Raise energy and delay fatigue during longer activities

10-20 grams of whey or casein protein 30-60 minutes pre-workout is optimal. Quickly absorbed whey is ideal for strength training while casein releases amino acids slowly to sustain endurance exercise.

Post-workout protein is crucial to:

- Rapidly initiate muscle repair and growth

- Replenish glycogen stores

- Blunt cortisol and reduce inflammation

Aim for 20-40 grams protein within 1 hour post-exercise. Whey, casein or blends provide fast digestion along with carbs to restore glycogen and facilitate recovery.

Properly timing protein around workouts potentiates performance gains. Let's look closer at maximizing amino acid availability...

Maximizing Amino Acid Availability and Uptake

Muscles can only grow and strengthen if amino acids from digested protein are delivered in sufficient amounts. Researchers propose the existence of an "anabolic window" post-exercise where muscles are primed for enhanced amino acid uptake and utilization.

Strategies to maximize amino acid availability and utilization include:

- **High leucine content** - The amino acid leucine directly stimulates muscle protein synthesis. Whey protein is naturally high in leucine.

- **Rapid protein digestion** - Quickly absorbed proteins like whey ensure fast amino acid spike.

- **Carb + protein combinations** - Adding carbs aids glycogen restoration, creating an optimal environment for amino acid uptake.

- **Frequent protein dosing** - Consuming protein every 3-5 hours maintains elevated amino acids between meals.

- **Slowing protein breakdown** - Creates steady influx of amino acids between meals to replace those lost from muscle breakdown during workouts.

Optimally timing high quality, rapidly digesting proteins that deliver key amino acids enhances the adaptive response to exercise.

Protein Timing for Strength vs Endurance Athletes

Protein's performance benefits differ slightly depending on training goals:

Strength athletes need more protein due to focus on muscle growth versus endurance athletes. Total daily protein should be in the range of:

- 0.7-1 g per lb bodyweight (or 150-200 g for a 200 lb athlete)

Pre- and post-workout protein is especially important on resistance training days:

- 20 g whey protein before workout

- 40 g whey + carb shake immediately after

Endurance athletes require relatively less daily protein but still more than sedentary individuals:

- 0.5 - 0.6 g per lb or 110-130 g for a 200 lb athlete

On higher mileage run or ride days:

- 20 g casein protein before exercise

- 20-30 g whey + carb protein after

Protein timing for both strength and endurance athletes focuses on optimizing amino acid availability to support differing metabolic demands depending on goals.

Protein for Faster Recovery

Vigorous training breaks down muscle tissue. Without adequate protein to provide amino acids for repair and rebuilding, muscles remain damaged, training adaptations are blunted, and performance suffers.

High protein intake enhances recovery by:

-Boosting post-workout muscle protein synthesis
-Reducing muscle protein breakdown -Replenishing glycogen stores
-Providing substrate for tissue repair -Reducing exercise induced muscle inflammation

Faster recovery allows for consistent, high-intensity training day after day and week after week. Active individuals should make protein a priority before, during and after exercise for optimal gains.

In summary, properly timing quality protein intake pre- and post-workout potentiates performance, accelerates muscle growth, minimizes soreness and catalyzes recovery.

Next let's explore the diverse benefits protein provides beyond athletics...

Chapter 6: Protein for Immunity, Bone Health, and Disease Prevention

While protein is crucial for athletes, its health benefits extend to everyone. Consuming adequate high-quality protein provides key advantages for immunity, bone health, and reducing risk of numerous age-related chronic diseases. We will examine:

- Protein and immune function

- Protein's benefits for bone matrix and fracture risk

- Associations between protein intake and longer lifespan

- Protein's role in preventing metabolic syndrome and diabetes

- Protein's antioxidant and anti-inflammatory effects

Appreciating protein's multifaceted benefits empowers you to take control of your health.

Protein Supports Immune Function

The immune system relies on adequate protein to function properly and protect against viruses, bacteria, and other pathogens.

Ways protein bolsters immunity:

- Producing antibodies requires amino acids from protein

- Key immune cells like lymphocytes need protein to grow and proliferate

- Making new immune cells following an immune challenge requires protein

- Secretory IgA antibodies in mucous to stop pathogens depends on protein

Those with protein deficiency are at increased risk of infections and longer duration of illness. Hospital patients with lower protein status have higher rates of acquired infections.

For optimized daily immune defense and resilience, include a source of high-quality protein at each meal.

Protein for Bone Health

Consuming adequate protein is crucial for building and maintaining strong, fracture-resistant bones.

Protein supports bone matrix formation by providing:

- Amino acids for producing collagen fibers

- Ingredients for crosslinking collagen strands

- Components of bone-mineralizing enzymes

Without sufficient protein, bone matrix production falters and osteoporosis risk climbs.

While excess protein was once feared to leach calcium from bones, newer evidence debunks this. Several meta-analyses find higher protein intake linked to:

- Increased bone mineral density

- Reduced bone loss with aging

- Decreased risk of hip fractures

- Faster recovery from fractures

Shoot for at least 30 g protein across three meals to reap benefits for bone integrity.

Protein and Longevity

Higher protein intake is associated with decreased mortality and increased lifespan across multiple studies.

In a 2018 analysis of over 13,000 adults followed for 32 years, participants ages 50-65 consuming the most protein had a:

- **29% lower risk of all-cause mortality**

- **28% reduced cardiovascular disease mortality**

Consuming protein beyond the RDA but within recommended limits supports healthy aging and longevity.

Reasons protein promotes lifespan include:

- Maintaining muscle mass

- Optimizing body composition

- Reducing chronic inflammation

- Preserving bone strength

- Supporting physical functioning

Adequate protein intake sustains health and vitality well into later decades of life.

Protein Defends Against Metabolic Disease

Eating more high-quality protein appears protective against obesity, diabetes, and metabolic syndrome.

In one study, doubling protein intake to 30% of calories reduced body fat gain by 60% and prevented insulin resistance.

Higher protein diets lower diabetes risk by:

- Improving insulin sensitivity

- Boosting satiety and weight control

- Reducing fat accumulation in the abdomen and liver

- Optimizing glucose regulation by the pancreas

- Slowing digestion to minimize blood sugar spikes

Substituting protein for refined carbs and low quality fats can help prevent metabolic disorders.

Protein's Antioxidant and Anti-Inflammatory Effects

High protein intake provides antioxidant and anti-inflammatory benefits vital for long-term health. Reasons include:

Glutathione Production

The amino acids cysteine and glycine needed to produce glutathione come from dietary protein. Glutathione is the body's master antioxidant, protecting cells against free radicals and oxidative stress.

Inflammation Reduction

Amino acids like arginine and glutamine help curb inflammatory pathways linked to disease development. Getting adequate protein reduces circulating inflammatory markers like CRP and interleukin-6.

Enhanced Detoxification

The liver needs quality protein to optimize production of cytochrome P450 enzymes vital for toxin elimination. This supports the body's natural detoxification processes.

Balanced Immune Function

Protein malnutrition can lead to improper immune system activation and excessive inflammation. Consuming adequate protein helps regulate balanced immune responses.

Lean Body Composition

Higher protein diets help reduce body fat, which directly decreases inflammatory adipokines. Leaner body composition is anti-inflammatory.

Optimizing your daily protein intake supports antioxidant status, immune balance, detoxification, and healthy aging free of chronic disease.

In summary, protein provides diverse and far-reaching benefits that encompass much more than just fitness goals. Prioritizing intake daily guards health on multiple fronts.

Now that you understand the varied benefits of protein, let's turn to determining your ideal protein intake...

Chapter 7: Finding Your Protein Sweet Spot

When it comes to daily protein needs, no one-size-fits-all rule applies. Optimal intake depends on individual factors like age, activity, health status and goals. This chapter provides guidance on:

- Estimating your protein requirements

- Signs you may need more (or less) protein

- Fine tuning intake for ideal health and function

- Incorporating high quality protein sources

Learning how to find your unique protein sweet spot provides a blueprint for utilizing protein's benefits discussed in previous chapters.

How Much Protein Do You Need?

The RDA for protein is 0.8 grams per kilogram of body weight or 0.36 grams per pound. This is the minimum required to prevent deficiency in 97.5% of people.

However, research indicates the RDA may not be ideal for optimal health, performance, disease prevention or metabolism.

Factors determining optimal protein needs include:

Age - Older adults need more protein to help maintain muscle mass and strength. The RDA may not meet needs after age 65.

Activity Level - Active individuals require more protein to support energy, performance and recovery. Sedentary people need less.

Condition/Disease - Illnesses like cancer, wounds or burns increase protein requirements for healing.

Weight Goals - Dieters need more protein to preserve lean mass when cutting calories. Athletes require more to build muscle.

Individual Variation - Subtle differences in metabolism, digestion and physiology affect ideal protein intake.

Considering these factors, optimal protein intake ranges are:

- **Sedentary people** - 0.5 to 0.7 g per pound of body weight

- **Active individuals** - 0.6 to 0.8 g per pound

- **Athletes** - 0.7 to 1.0 g per pound

- **Elderly** - 0.7 to 1.0 g per pound

- **Pregnant/nursing** - 0.7 to 1.0 g per pound

The upper end of each range maximizes protein's benefits while staying within safe limits, allowing room for individual variation.

Let's look at signs you may need more (or less) protein.

Signs You May Need More Protein

Here are signs you may benefit from increasing your protein intake:

- Unintentional muscle loss or weakness

- Poor recovery from exercise

- Inadequate satiety and frequent cravings

- Fatigue, low energy and brain fog

- High BMI but little muscle definition

- Poor wound healing and frequent illness

- Hair loss or brittle/peeling nails

- Blood sugar swings and sugar cravings

- Loss of libido or sexual function

Ramping up daily protein by 20-30 grams can help resolve these issues if low intake is the cause. Spread extra protein across meals and snacks.

Signs You Need Less Protein

Here are signs you may be getting too much protein:

- Kidney problems or gout

- Dehydration and electrolyte imbalances

- High ammonia levels

- Weight gain from overconsuming calories

- Constipation

- Fatigue or headaches

- Mood issues like anxiety or irritation

- Insomnia

- Bloating and indigestion

If these arise, try reducing daily protein intake by 20-30 grams for 2-3 weeks and monitor changes. Drink plenty of non-caffeinated fluids and increase fiber to alleviate potential side effects.

Fine Tuning Your Intake

Track your current protein intake by recording foods and beverages for 3-5 days. Calculate average grams consumed.

Compare your current intake to the optimal range for your demographic and goals. Are you above, at, or below your ideal protein target?

If below, incorporate more high-quality protein sources into meals and snacks. Ramp up gradually in 10-20 gram increments. Reassess in 2-3 weeks.

If already at or above your goal, you may not need adjustments. But be mindful of any signs of excess noted above.

Individualize fine tuning based on changes in body composition, energy, cravings, exercise recovery etc. Determine the amount that helps you feel and perform at your best.

Incorporating Quality Protein Sources

Focus on high quality proteins with good digestibility and PDCAAS scores:

Animal Proteins: Eggs, Greek yogurt, cottage cheese, whey, casein, milk, fish, chicken, beef, pork

Plant Proteins: Soy, seitan, tempeh, edamame, quinoa, lentils, beans, nuts, seeds

Protein Supplements: Whey, casein, collagen, egg white protein, pea, rice, hemp blends

Aim for a variety to obtain all the essential amino acids. Spread protein intake evenly throughout the day for optimal muscle protein synthesis.

Finding your protein sweet spot takes some personal experimentation. Be observant of how increased protein intake affects your energy, body composition, workouts, cravings and other health parameters. Enjoy the journey to uncovering your ideal protein needs!

Conclusion

If you've made it this far, congratulations on expanding your protein knowledge. You now understand the diverse and far-reaching roles protein plays in health, performance, disease prevention and longevity.

This book has taken you on a journey through protein's effects on metabolism, weight loss, immunity, bone health, energy levels, muscle building, and recovery. You've learned the ins and outs of protein quality, timing, and differences between animal and plant sources. We've covered how to determine and fine tune your individual protein needs based on your unique goals and activity levels.

Armed with this protein wisdom, you have the tools to harness protein's incredible power. Let's recap some of the key points:

Protein powers life - As the very building blocks of cells and tissues, proteins drive virtually every biological process in the body. Getting adequate high-quality protein should be non-negotiable.

Pay attention to timing - When you eat protein matters. Distributing intake throughout the day supports satiety, muscle synthesis and stable energy. Pre- and post-workout protein optimizes performance and recovery.

Focus on quality sources - Complete proteins from animal foods or properly combined plant proteins ensure you get all the essential amino acids. Lean meats, dairy, eggs, whey and well-balanced plant proteins are excellent choices.

Protein protects health - Higher protein diets are linked to lower risks of obesity, osteoporosis, diabetes, heart disease and premature death. Protein also boosts immunity and antioxidant status.

Protein preserves muscle mass - Consuming adequate high-quality protein helps maintain metabolism by reducing age- and diet-related muscle loss while supporting gains in athletes.

Individualize your intake - While the RDA of 0.8 g/kg provides a minimum requirement, optimal protein needs depend on your unique lifestyle, body composition and health status. More active individuals need more.

Experiment and track - Try adjusting your protein intake gradually while monitoring energy, cravings, body composition and workouts. Track your diet to determine your ideal protein sweet spot.

The central message is that making high-quality protein a priority provides incredible benefits for your health, body, performance and peace of mind. But protein can only work its magic if you give it the opportunity.

Start Unlocking Protein's Potential

Don't just take this book's word for it - put the protein strategies into practice in your own life:

- **Incorporate more lean proteins** - Try new protein preparations and sources to eat a wider variety.

- **Time protein intake** - Spread protein throughout the day and pre/post workouts.

- **Select high quality sources** - Emphasize proteins with high bioavailability and PDCAAS scores.

- **Adjust your protein intake** - Gradually increase your daily protein if below optimal targets.

- **Track changes** - Note effects on energy, cravings, body composition, strength etc.

- **Read labels** - Choose foods with higher protein-to-carb ratios.

- **Mitigate deficiencies** - Combine plant proteins or use supplements if needed.

- **Stay hydrated** - Drink adequate water and reduce sodium to support kidney function.

- **Be patient** - Allow 2-3 weeks to notice changes from altered protein intake.

Stick with the changes for a few months to reap sustained benefits on your health, appearance, performance and peace of mind.

Parting Words

This book has illuminated the diverse and compelling evidence demonstrating protein's ability to transform health. From profound roles in weight management, metabolism and muscle building to reducing disease risk and supporting immunity and bone health, protein delivers.

Yet protein can only work its magic if you give it the chance. Many people sabotage themselves with suboptimal low protein diets. I hope this book has convinced you to make high-quality protein a priority in your food selections.

Approach protein not as just another nutrient, but as an indispensable dietary foundation without which good health crumbles. I encourage you to experiment, get creative, be consistent and unlock protein's monumental potential in your own life. Just imagine how good your health, body and performance can feel when protein is optimized.

The journey begins with your next bite - now that you understand protein's importance, it's time to fuel your cells properly. I wish you the very best as you leverage protein to transform your health and reach new heights of energy, strength and vitality. Be sure to share your protein victories with me!

About the Author

Omolola Habib is a down-to-earth naturopathic doctor, certified health coach, and proud protein enthusiast on a mission to revolutionize health, one bite at a time.

As a naturopathic physician, Omolola brings a holistic lens to wellness. She understands the body as an interconnected system, recognizing how small changes in diet and lifestyle can create big shifts in health.

Omolola's passion is empowering people to take charge of their own vitality. She knows that lasting change starts from within, which is why she offers practical, personalized guidance to help clients discover what works best for their unique bodies.

While she draws on her strong foundation in natural medicine, Omolola realizes no one diet fits all. Her approach is flexible and collaborative. She motivates people through support rather than strict rules.

In writing "Unlocking the Power of Protein," Omolola distills decades of clinical experience and the latest scientific research into an actionable roadmap. More than a book, it's an invitation to revolutionize your own health journey through the power of protein.

Omolola firmly believes small steps cultivate big change. She wrote this book to cut through the confusion around protein and offer simple, flexible strategies anyone can integrate. Because she knows when people feel empowered in their health, anything is possible!